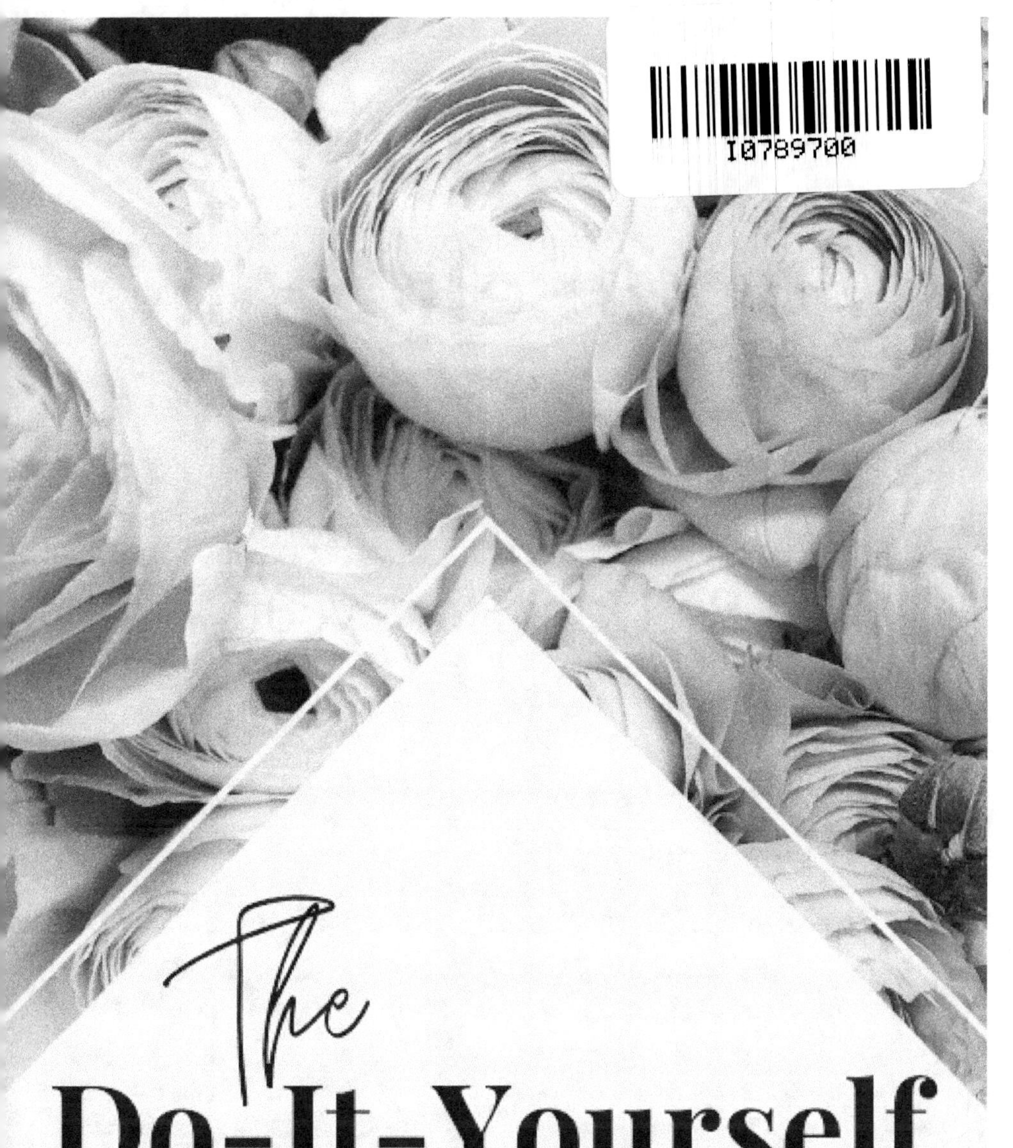

The
Do-It-Yourself
Skin Care
Manual

DANI HONEYCUTT

The Do-It-Yourself Skin Care Manual

By Dani Honeycutt

DISCLAIMER:

This information is not presented by a medical practitioner and is for educational and informational purposes only. The content is not intended to be a substitute for professional medical advice, diagnosis, or treatment. Always seek the advice of your physician or other qualified healthcare provider with any questions you may have regarding a medical condition. Never disregard professional medical advice or delay in seeking it because of something you have read.

Table of Contents

FOREWORD

This has been a journey years in the making. Both publishing my first book and falling in love with the way my face looks naturally. I have battled years with cystic acne from PCOS, scarring, hyperpigmentation, eczema, excessive dry skin, rashes, rosacea and so much more.

As a pimple-prone high school girl, I used to think that just a bar of soap…yes, the one I also washed my body with…was good enough to wash my face with. My dry skin issue started then as well.

I remember getting up and scrubbing my face with a Samp washcloth until all the dry skin was gone from around my mouth. In fact, I would scrub so hard that often times I would take off healthy skin as well. That resulted in raw and sometimes bleeding patches around my mouth. I felt horrible and disgusting. I would try to pile on drug store makeup to cover up my raw skin.

I do not think there was a single day in my high school career that I went to school without makeup on. Of course, I rarely washed my makeup off before I went to bed for the night. It was an endless cycle of breakouts and dry skin.

Fast forward to my late twenties when I really started to take care of my skin. I started digging in to all of these fancy and expensive skin care regimens. I have known my entire life that I have sensitive skin. One of them resulted in slight burns on my face! Not all skincare chemicals are created equally.

I made sure that I was removing any makeup that I had worn before I went to sleep for the night. My face continued to blister with cystic acne. Touching my face to even wash it was so painful during these times.

Right before I turned thirty, I found out that I have PCOS, which is polycystic ovary syndrome. It causes massive hormonal imbalance and effects my health in various ways, one of which is cystic acne.

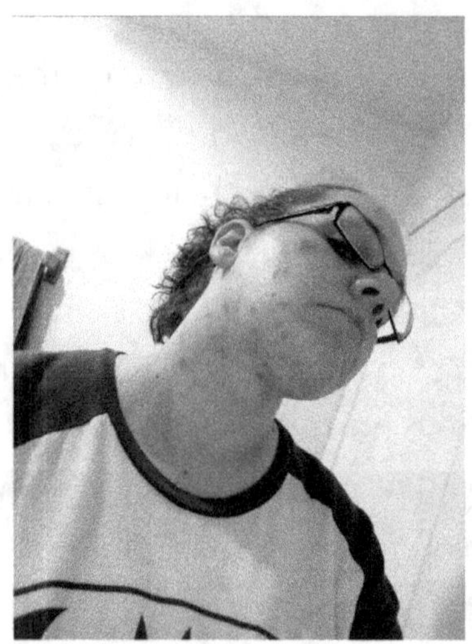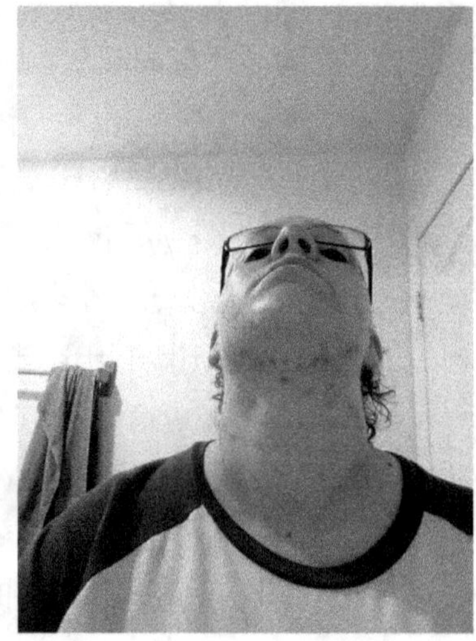

I can remember standing in front of the mirror in my fiancé's apartment in tears. It was so painful, but the way I felt about myself was even more painful. I continued to try to get my acne under control, while I worked with the doctor on my health.

Over the past five years, I have finally found products that do not aggravate my skin or cause burning from chemicals. It's been in front of my face the whole times. The answer was natural products. I am still working on my health and have since been diagnosed with autoimmune disease. Health is just as important for our face as a skincare routine.

Our skin is our largest organ. Learning to take care of your skin will help combat some of your skincare woes, such as fine lines and wrinkles. Since using more natural products and creating a skincare routine that I can stick to, my face has changed dramatically!

I hope that you benefit from this book and the information within. If you choose to implement any of the information in this book, please feel free to share your results on social media and include #HoneyDBeauty

Thank you for spending your time learning from me. I can not wait to connect with you and become friends. Enjoy!

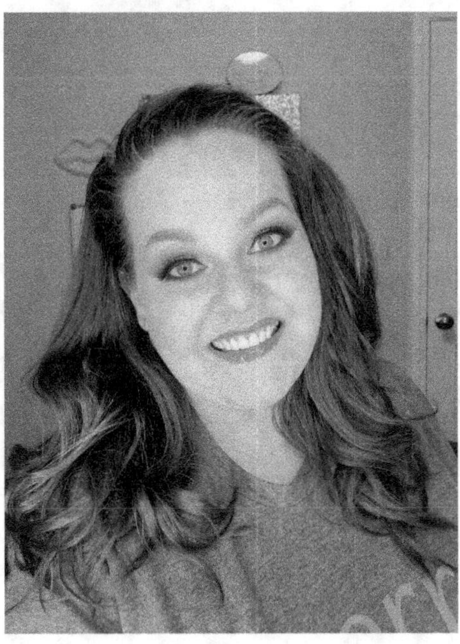

DO IT YOURSELF SKIN CARE MANUAL

In a world of tight schedules, harmful pollution, chemically-laden products, high anxiety, and environmental toxin overload, it is impossible for our skin not to feel and show the effects of it all! Thankfully, with a little commitment, you can maintain your skin's natural beauty in the comfort of your own home! Keep reading to get some tips and simple at-home methods to reduce stress, maintain your radiant skin, and decrease the signs of aging!

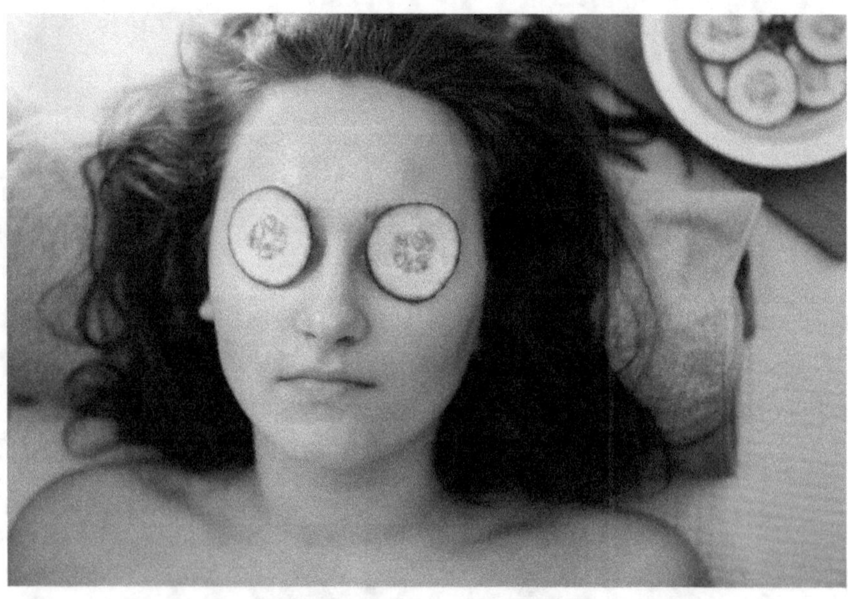

CLEANSING YOUR SKIN

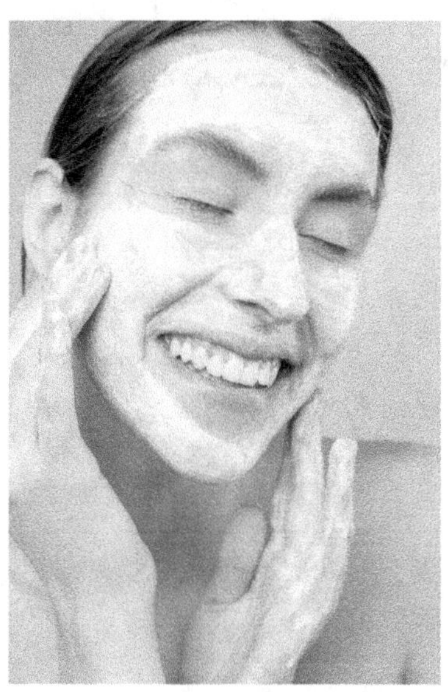

The first step in caring for your skin is to properly cleanse it! Perspiration, grease, dust, stale make-up, dirt, and bacteria all collect on your skin and must be completely removed. There are many different skin types; oily, dry, sensitive, and prone to acne. Different cleansers do better with each individual type based on the pH and other varying factors. Cleansing helps to clean the skin, open the pores, and allows for the skin to best absorb the products you are going to apply. If you wear a good amount of make-up, you may want to first use a makeup remover to get the majority of the make-up off your face prior to cleansing.

To properly cleanse, begin by wetting the face with lukewarm water. Apply the cleanser that is best for your skin type on your face and neck and gently massage in a circular, upward motion for at least five minutes (duration also depends on the instructions provided with the cleanser you are using). Remove by using a damp washcloth and warm water to ensure all of the residue is removed from the face.

TONING YOUR SKIN

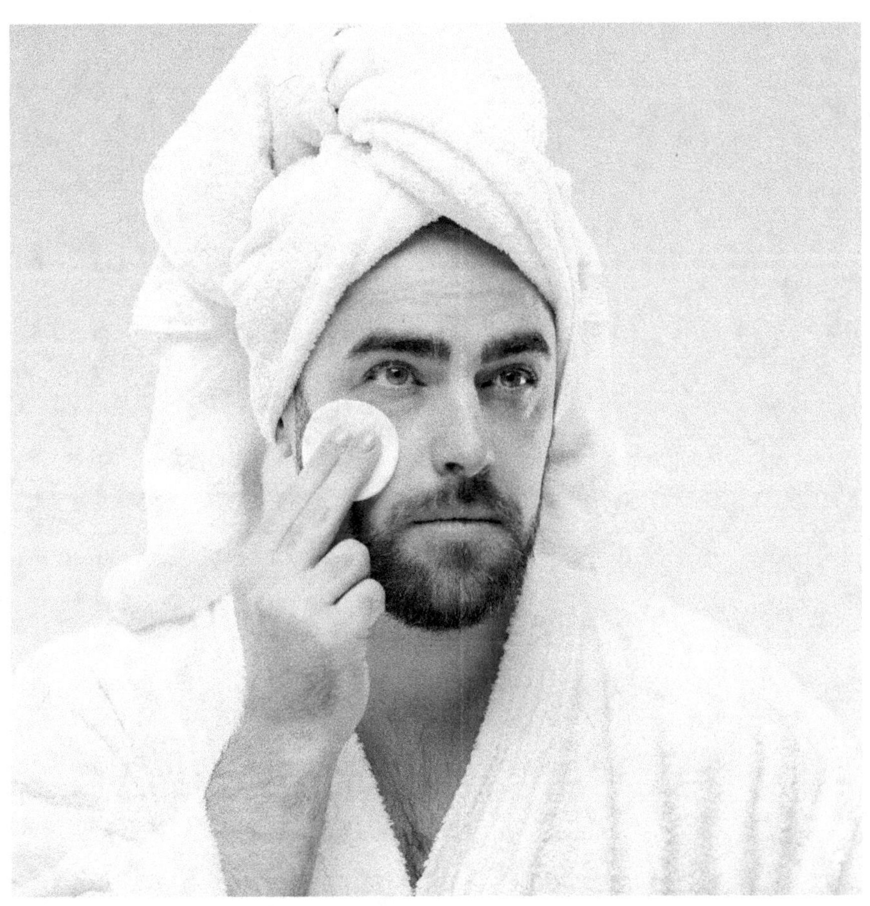

Next, tone your skin using skin freshener (mild), skin tonic (medium strength), or an astringent lotion (strong). Toning is important because it helps remove any remaining greasiness on your skin after the cleansing process is complete. It helps to close pores and maintain the skin's natural pH, and if you intend to use makeup, it leaves a smooth clean texture which will hold foundation and powder much longer.

NOURISHING YOUR SKIN

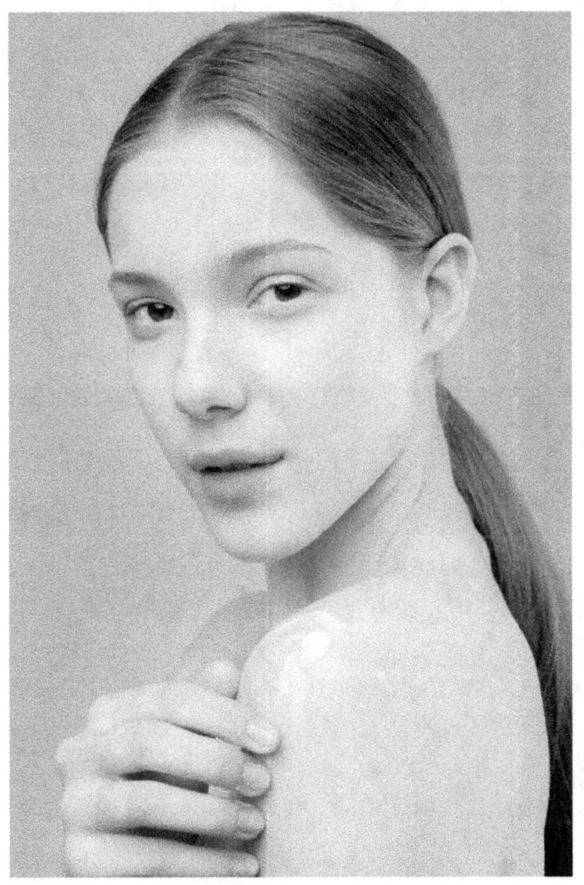

Nourishing your skin is also an essential part of any beauty routine. Dirt, dust, hot and cold weather, cosmetics, and even sunlight, all tend to dry out the skin, robbing it of moisture and oil. Consequently, making sure to cleanse your face each night before bed is essential to younger looking skin. Skin "foods" or moisturizers attempt to replenish nourishment to the skin, reviving its natural healthiness. Again, different moisturizers work well for different skin types. If your skin is more on the oily side, avoid moisturizers that contain oils and opt for one that contains glycerin instead. If you have drier skin, applying a moisturizer right after washing your face is beneficial to prevent drying and to get moisturizer locked in right away. If you have neutral skin, you can usually get away with using a product that contains oil or glycerin. Just make sure to look for a product for neutral skin types.

FACIAL

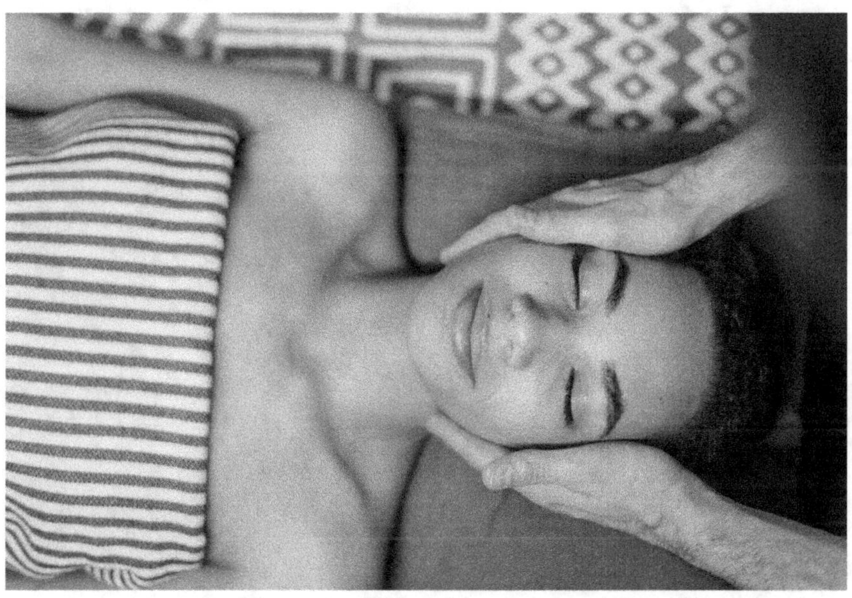

A facial is the quickest way of cleansing, reviving, and brightening faded skin, leaving the skin light, soft and glowing. A facial also does a thorough job of relaxing frazzled nerves so that you emerge not only looking younger but also feeling fresher and more relaxed! A facial once or twice each month will ensure rejuvenated and fresh skin for a long time to come!

If it is in your budget to seek out a spa or professional for your facial, find someone who uses natural products and pays attention to your skin type. However, if you do not have the time or cannot afford the luxury of regular salon treatments, you can give yourself a facial at home! Choose a time when you can be undisturbed and quiet, and get everything ready before you start so that you can relax and really enjoy it!

AT-HOME FACIAL

Follow the routine below for a quick, at-home facial:

- Tie your hair away from your face and neck, using a headband to pull any remaining hair away from your forehead.

- Begin by removing your makeup either using makeup remover wipes, coconut oil or another method to remove all residue from the face. Cleanse your face and neck with a good cleanser and thoroughly remove.

- The next step is a gentle exfoliation to remove dead skin cells, dirt, and bacteria allowing the skin to best absorb the other products. We love using a simple, DIY exfoliant of organic coffee grounds, hot water, and warmed organic coconut oil but you can also find wonderful store-bought products to use.

- Prepare a face mask suited to your skin type. On a thoroughly cleansed and exfoliated face, spread a fairly thick layer avoiding the mouth area and creating large circles round the eyes. Then, lie on your back and keep the mask on for 15 to 20 minutes or until dry. There are many options for creating an amazing mask at home but the one we love the most is a simple concoction of organic coconut oil, honey and fresh avocado.

- When the mask is dry, wash your face and neck with lukewarm water, keeping your eyes closed. Dry your skin and apply your favorite toner that is best for your skin type.

- Lastly, now that the skin is thoroughly cleansed, exfoliated, and the pores are open, it is time to apply skin serum and/or moisturizer to the face. Spend some time massaging it in using upward, circular motions.

MASSAGING YOUR SKIN

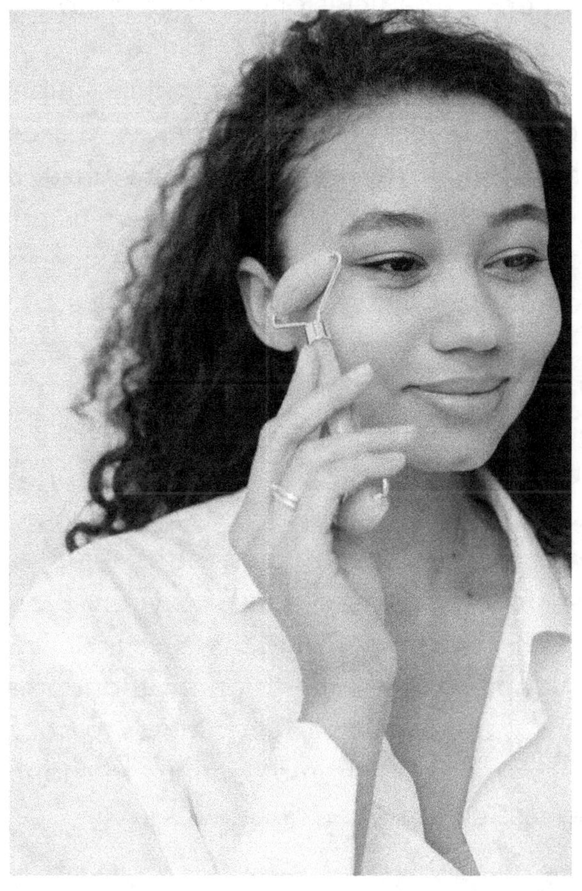

Massaging your face is another essential practice for healthy skin and can also be really relaxing! While being an effective way to counter wrinkles, massaging is a slow process and its results are obvious only if it is practiced regularly for an extended period of time. That said, there is no doubt that massage is highly beneficial for tightening facial tissues, increasing blood flow, stimulating nerves and thus, boosting collagen production.

Massage is most effective if the skin is thoroughly cleansed first. Do not forget to remove all traces of makeup, otherwise particles of dirt will end up blocking the pores of the skin. If the skin is oily, then remove oiliness by applying cleansing milk or some astringent lotion. Fresh lemon juice is also very effective in removing excess oiliness. If the skin is dry, use a good moisturizer before massaging it. Finally, apply Vitamin E cream using only enough to give sufficient greasiness to the skin so that the hands and fingers move smoothly on the face.

After having cleaned the skin, press it with light but firm fingers, putting a little pressure while applying a good moisturizer. Make sure to hold the skin firmly and apply even pressure. The massage should start from the neck and move upwards ending at the forehead or temples. Veins and tissues get an increased flow of oxygen/ blood supply by this process. The skin around the eyes is delicate so it is advisable to apply cream on this part without pressing it in too deeply. Cream takes 15 to 20 minutes to get absorbed by the skin, so massage should continue that long. Gently wipe off excess cream when finished.

THE ART OF MASSAGING

- Slow Massage - This is the most common method of massage and the most relaxing. The secret is to massage slowly while patting the skin. Using the fleshy part of your finger tips, press the skin lightly with a slow, stroking motion.. The process starts at the base of the neck at a slow speed. Stroking gives rest to the nerves and the vibration is useful in subduing pain that might be caused over more sensitive areas..

- Fast Massage - The front half of both the palms are used to massage at speed, taking care to make a circular motion upwards

- Pressure Massage - This is a method when slow, deep pressure is applied by the fingertips and is very effective for removing pouches beneath eyes.

-Stroking Massage - Cheeks are stroked with the tips of fingers and strokes are applied from the nose to the temples on both sides

- Pinching Massage - Effective for a sagging chin or wrinkles on the jawline, the skin is held, as in pinchers, between the thumb and fingers and gently massaged.

* Friction Massage - This massage requires pressure on the skin while it is being moved over the underlying bone and muscle structures. Fingers or palms are usually best for this type of massage and hard movements are usually employed on the scalp while light movements are used on the face and neck.

* Piano Playing Movements - This exercise develops facial muscles and makes them firm. It should be done with the fingers on the entire face, especially the cheek area.

MAKING YOUR OWN SKIN PRODUCTS

- *DIY Face Scrub*

In a bowl combine 1/2 cup of Organic Brown Sugar and 1/4 cup of Organic Avocado Oil. Mix well until combined. Scoop out a kiwi, muddle it down and then mix it in with the sugar and oil. Store the mixture in an air-tight glass jar and refrigerate for up to two weeks.

- *Handmade Massage Oil*

Add 1/4 cup of your favorite carrier oil to a jar or container(almond oil, avocado oil, or coconut oil are all great options) Next, choose your favorite essential oil or combination of oils and add 1 tsp total to the carrier oil. Mix well and allow to stand overnight.

- *Anti-wrinkle Cream*

Melt together 2 tablespoons lanolin or beeswax, 2 tablespoons almond oil and 1 tablespoon apricot oil. Then add 3 tablespoons lemon juice or lemon essential oil. Apricots are very rich in vitamin A and this mixture is great for helping to reduce wrinkles!

- *Anti-wrinkle Lotion*

Mix together the following ingredients: 1/4 cup of shea butter, 1 tbsp coconut or almond oil, and 16 drops of your favorite essential oil (we love lavender, rosemary, frankincense, and lemon). Mix well by hand or in a mixer and add to a clean jar.

MY FAVORITE PRODUCTS

I love to double cleanse using oil based cleansers. Since some makeup has an oil base, I need an oil to remove the makeup from my pores. My two favorite oil based cleansers are Fourth Ray BFD Oil Cleanser and Fourth Ray AM to the PM Gel Cleanser. Both of these cleansers can be found at http://www.colourpop.com

As a toner, I am head over heels for all natural rose water. I make this at home myself. Using rose petals, distilled water, aloe vera and a few other items. The aloe vera helps soothe irritated skin while the rose uplifts.

I use a few different serums. An installs serum, a face serum, and an eye serum. All three of these serums are inspired and centered around the powerful properties found in the Swiss Red Love Apple which contain extraordinary antioxidants, among other benefits. The apple stem cells are some of the distinct ingredients that power our proprietary anti-aging products. They can be found at https://www.everra.com/store/honeydbeauty/product-category/skincare/

I use a rose quartz facial roller and gua sha that I purchased as a kit from Amazon for massage and circulation.

For nourishment, I use the Fourth Ray The Daily Face Cream. It's packed with plant-derived ingredients and my skin soaks it up. It can be found at http://www.colourpop.com

So there you have it! By following these simple tips, and being consistent with your routines, you can easily start having brighter, healthier, and more rejuvenated looking skin in no time at all!

For more products that I love to use that are natural and cruelty-free visit http://www.everra.com/store/honeydbeauty

For more info on health and wellness visit http://honeydbeauty.com

ABOUT THE AUTHOR

Dani lives in east Tennessee with her husband, Jonathan, and their chi-weenie, Tulip. Jonathan and Dani have been happily married for 5 years. Due to her health, Dani is unable to have children. She spends her time cuddling with her dog, who loves every moment.

Dani loves to teach and help others with their beauty and wellness needs in a holistic way. She is currently studying to become a certified health and wellness coach, as well as a life coach.

Dani has been writing for several years, which included years as a journalist for a local newspaper. She left the newspaper industry to become an entrepreneur. She now owns a beauty and wellness company, HoneyDBeauty. She helps others start their own beauty and wellness business, and works with customers to help match them with products that help them.

For more information about Dani, please visit http://honeydbeauty.com

Follow Dani on Facebook http://www.facebook.com/daniddyer

Follow Dani on Instagram http://www.instagram.com/danidyer